Oikonomics
Because Home is Everywhere You Are

Creating comfortable spaces in all places
home, office and beyond!

Deidre Ann Johnson
Massage Therapist
Physical Therapist
Certified Ergonomic Assessment Specialist
Certified Pilates Instructor

New York, New York
2017

Printed in the United States of America

First Printing, 2018

Createspace Publishing
Columbia, SC

www.Oikonomics.net

Dedication

This book is dedicated to the memory of my Dad, Robert T. Johnson who loved his family more than life itself.

I miss you much.

Acknowledgements

Many thanks to all of the people who inspire and encourage me to grow to greater heights each and every day and without whom this book might not be:

My father, Robert Johnson who always supported the gazillion things I've done in my life;

Lynette Johnson, the best sister in the world, who never ceases to give honest feedback whether I've asked for it or not; my brother through marriage, Gerry, for his hilarity; my nephews Jared and Matthew for being so awesome!

Stella McKeown for her immense talent and patience editing this book;

Harold McKeown for his amazing vision and ability to see not one, two or three but five and six steps ahead. Who has continued to encourage me to achieve more so I can have an answer to his question, "So…what's next?" "What you been up to?" And who, by the way, makes GREAT Manhattans!!

To Richard McKeown, my partner in life, who continues to encourage me by way of example…say yes to everything and then figure it out.

Sheila (Sheila Gyrl) Prevost, artist extraordinaire. Thank you for your branding expertise and your willingness to brainstorm ideas with me to help me clarify my vision.

My dear friends, Walter Holland and Howard Frey for additional editorial suggestions for this book and brainstorming ideas.

Adriana Ramirez, my fellow wine enthusiast, for her support and encouragement.

In working with my patients or massage therapy clients, I realized that those coming to me with non-traumatic events (traumatic events being a fall or surgery) complained mostly about the same things—back pain, neck and shoulder pain, wrist and elbow pain. They were all desk jockeys glued to their computers from sun up to sun down, rarely taking breaks during the day for themselves.

I also realized that it wasn't specific to the physical confines of their brick and mortar office spaces. These days, many people telecommunicate from the comfort (and I use that word with a hint of sarcasm) of their own homes.

As I queried about their work spaces at home, my mind was blown. Here are some examples:

- "I usually lay in bed with my laptop resting on my belly;"
- "My laptop is on a TV stand while I sit on the couch;"
- "I work on my kitchen counter top while sitting on a bar stool
- "I'm on the couch with the laptop on my lap."

Can you understand what's wrong with the above scenarios? Do you see how sitting for hours in positions that absolutely do not support muscular balance and promote stiffness can ultimately result in chronic pain? PLEEEASSSE tell me you do!!!

We live in a world where we can be plugged-in 24/7/365 (why anyone would want to be attached in this way is beyond me). The work must get done or the world will fall off its axis and we will all be doomed!!!

It's the rat race on steroids. And guess what? The work doesn't ever stop, even when you clear your desk. You get to come back and do it again and again and again.

AHHHHHHH. Take time for yourself. Pay attention to what your body is telling you, it's smarter than our minds are, trust me on that. Stretch. Breathe…deeply. Walk. Drink more water and less coffee. Come back to your desk with more clarity and ideas. Take two minutes to go to your most happy place for inspiration. Meditate for 30 seconds. The work will still be there waiting for you and you will be in a better place physically, emotionally and spiritually to get it done without causing harm to yourself in the process.

Apply this concept to all areas of your life. Driving, flying, practicing your instrument. It doesn't matter. Take a breather. You will be better for it, I promise.

Table of Contents

W e are all very familiar with ergonomics - *Ergon* from the Greek words meaning work and *Nomos* meaning law. The purpose of ergonomics is to apply certain principles or laws to the way we work in order to promote our biomechanical safety, efficiency, effectiveness and endurance. In other words it's a process which fits the workplace to the worker thereby reducing stress, fatigue and injury.

The history of ergonomics, though not the word, pre-dates the industrial revolution. The goal of ergonomics has always been to do things differently and more easily in order to reduce the level of physical and emotional stress. It can be traced as far back as early man who made tools from pebbles and bones and fashioned them in a way that made tasks easier.

In the 16th century, Dr. Bernardino Ramazinni correlated patient injuries with their occupations and work environments and compiled his findings into a medical journal entitled, "De Morbis Artificum" (Diseases of Workers). It was with these writings that the foundation for ergonomics was laid.

The word "ergonomics" however, did not appear for another 200 years. In 1857, it was created and used by Wojciech Jastrzebowski in a narrative he had written about the science of nature.

In 1911, a monograph entitled "The Principles of Scientific Management" was written by Frederick Winslow Taylor. Taylor was an American manufacturing manager, mechanical engineer and in later years a management consultant. In this monograph, he detailed how to increase the efficacy of a worker by improving the process of the task. For example, Taylor realized that by reducing the weight and size of coal shovels, the amount of coal being shoveled by workers could be tripled. These ideas lead to reduced work injuries and an increase in production levels.

Also in the 1900s, Frank and Lillian Gilbreth expanded Taylor's methods and came up with the "Time and Motion Studies." They looked at the different techniques that would help reduce the amount of unnecessary motions required to perform a specific task. The study helped reduce the number of motions required in bricklaying which allowed bricklayers to increase productivity from 120 up to 350 bricks an hour. With these studies, ergonomics became a legitimate discipline.

Would you believe me if I told you that WWII also utilized ergonomics? During this war, it was noted that aircrafts in good condition and flown by the best pilots still had a high crash rate. An army officer, Alphonse Chapanis, had the idea to reduce pilot errors by replacing confusing designs in airplane cockpits with more logical controls.

I have developed what I have termed Oikonomics from the Greek word *Oikos* meaning home and *Nomos* meaning law. Why Oikonomics?

Because home is EVERYWHERE you are--whether it's in your actual home, at work or in the car. It is important to be aware of your posture no matter what you are doing, especially if you are performing an activity for a prolonged period of time (longer than 30 mins).

Oikonomics is about being present in your body, listening to what your muscles are telling you. Being aware of tension—are your shoulders up by your ears? Are you knitting your brow? Gritting your teeth? Do you chest breathe vs. breathing diaphragmatically? I will teach you techniques to tap into areas of tension and make adjustments accordingly. Taking the time to read and apply them now will save you time and money in rehabilitation later to alleviate a chronic musculoskeletal disorder (MSD).

The easiest thing to do when you are feeling tense is to MOVE! That's what our bodies are meant to do. Studies suggest that even with the recommended 30 mins of exercise 3 days a week, sedentary lifestyles during work and recreation can have serious health implications including type 2 diabetes, obesity and cardiovascular disease.

When at work, every thirty minutes, get up and
S -T- R- E -T - C - H. Walk around (I'm sure there's an app for
that!). Blood and oxygen will surge through your muscles
rejuvenating you and giving you clarity of thought which brings new
ideas. Your brain is a muscle too!

W ork is definitely home; at least for the 8 - 14 hours that you are there. Your attention is splintered in various directions and the last thing you think about is yourself. You don't realize that your neck and shoulders are tense, that your back is tight or that your teeth are clenched. It's not until you come home from work that EVERYTHING hurts. Here are some basic things you need to put in place to make things a little better:

You
- Head level or slightly downward in regards to your line of sight for the activity at hand
- Shoulders relaxed
- Elbows at sides about 90 degrees
- Sit upright or slightly reclining
- Low back supported
- Keep wrists straight (+/- 15 degrees)
- Keep knees at or below hip level; no pressure on the back of knees
- Feet out in front and supported

Workstation

Chair

This is one of your most important choices because this is the surface you are in contact with the most. Take into account your height. If you are taller or shorter, there are chairs that accommodate for that.

- Lumbar support - Some chairs come with an adjustable lumbar support; nice, but not a deal breaker if you don't have one.
- Padded arms, (adjustable & removable) - Hard surfaces can create contact distress to soft tissue which is why having padded arms is a benefit.
- Adjustability - Ensures that your arms are resting in the correct biomechanically neutral position and that the height and tilt of chair can be modified.

All backrests should support your lumbar spine and allow clearance for your buttocks.

- If you require upper body mobility, a low back rest (below the shoulder blades) would be best so as not to interfere with arm movement.
- Like to recline? A tall backrest would serve your purpose. Make sure that you still feel support in your low back area.
- Waterfall front edge - A waterfall edge slopes down in the front providing a softer surface.
- Easy to reach controls - If they are easy to reach, you are more likely to use them to make yourself more comfortable.
- 5 caster base - Provides stability.
- Chair depth adjustment - An adjustable seat pan will prevent contact between the edge of the chair and the back of your knees. A 2 to 3 inch distance is adequate.
- Keyboard/keyboard tray - There are fancy split keyboards that will allow a more natural position for your wrists while typing. But the more important thing to do is to take frequent stretch breaks to relax your muscles. If you have a keyboard tray, there should be adequate space between it and your knees.

Monitor placement and tilt

- The monitor should be at arm's length directly in front of you at eye level or slightly below.

Document Holder

- USE A DOCUMENT HOLDER!! This will prevent excessive head/neck flexion/extension/rotation from document to monitor. It should be placed in front of you or on the side of your dominant eye.

> *How to find your dominant eye*
> *With both eyes open, make a triangle with the index fingers and thumbs of both hands. Look through the triangle and center something such as a doorknob in the triangle. Close your left eye. If the object remains in view, you are right eye dominant. If closing your right eye keeps the object in view, you are left eye dominant.*

Glare

- To prevent glare, place monitors at 90 degree angles of windows or directly under overhead lights. If you can't control that, get an anti-glare screen.

Lap tops - Great for mobility. Bad for posture. If you must use one at work, use a detachable keyboard. Do everything you can to maintain a neutral position while working.

Phones

- Don't hold the phone between your ear and your neck...*please!!* This is the number one reason why people have neck and shoulder pain and they NEVER understand WHY in the world their neck hurts. Do you walk around during your day with your head tilted way over to your shoulder??

Mouse

- There are many ergonomic mouses **(mice??)** on the market. One of the easiest ways to prevent overuse is to place the mouse on your less dominant side (a great way to create more neural synapses as your brain learns to use the weaker hand). The other way to prevent overuse? Get up and move. Stretch your wrist muscles, shake your hands.

Work zone - Your work zone is divided into two functional areas.
1. *Primary work zone. This is your forward reach for frequent usage items, measured 16 inches from the edge of your workspace.*

2. *Secondary work zone. This is your forward reach for occasional usage items, measured 24 inches from the edge of your workspace.*

However, even if you correctly implement all of the above and are awarded **Work Station of the Year,** you will STILL suffer from repetitive stress injuries if you don't *MOVE!* I cannot emphasize this enough but will try to.

Every 15 minutes change your body position. Every 30 minutes actually get up out of your chair and stretch, yawn, get a drink of water or use the rest room to splash your face with cool refreshing water. Below are some stretches you should do at work:

Every 15 minutes:
- Unweight your butt from the chair
- Toes up/toes down

Every 30 minutes:
- Fingers - open and close your fingers, bring some blood to those digits.
- Wrist flexors - place your hands together as in prayer in front of your nose. Bring your hands down to the middle of your chest. You will feel a nice stretch of your flexors.
- Wrist extensors - Bring your arm out in front of you with your fingers pointed down. Use your other hand to apply a gentle pressure to your downward facing fingers towards you. You will feel a nice stretch to your extensors.
- Shoulders - Bring one arm across your chest. Use your other hand to apply pressure to your elbow to give a gentle stretch. Repeat other side.
- Shoulder blade retractions - Squeeze your shoulder blades together 10 times.
- Shoulder blade depressions - Drop your arms to your sides. Reach your fingers towards the floor. Repeat 10 times.
- Neck stretch - Bring your right ear to your right shoulder, hold 30 seconds. Keep same position and now look down towards your right hip. Hold for 30 seconds. Repeat other side.
- Chin tucks - Make a double chin. Relax. Repeat 10 times.
- Backward bends - Stand up. Place your hands on your hips and gently lean backwards. Return to starting position. Repeat 5 times.

I got to thinking about this at work. I had a patient who complained of neck pain. I treated him and he got better. During the course of treatment we talked about his work station and a few minor improvements that could be made but honestly, it wasn't that bad. So off he went back to his life, his neck feeling better.

A few months later he returned with the same problem. What changed? Nothing really, the neck just began to hurt again. There had to be some reason why but what was it? He had no idea.

We began treatment - soft tissue release, range of motion, manual traction. During this we were talking. At some point we talked about television and out of the blue he said, "You know what? My television is mounted up on the wall and when I watch it I'm looking up. I think that's why my neck hurts."

Brilliant. Body positioning and posture are not only important at work; they are important at home as well. *Especially* at home because that's where we're the most comfortable and least likely to pay attention to how we're sitting, lying, lounging in our space. It's like when you've been driving for quite a distance and you're almost home. Almost home is when you have to be the most vigilant because you slip into autopilot and stop paying attention. This is when car accidents commonly occur.

There's lounging and there's lounging smart which will actually ensure that you are more comfortable with less opportunity for joint stiffness, aches and pains.

Furniture

Couches and Chairs
We think couches and chairs should be big and squishy so much so that when you sit down in them you sink about a foot. Not true. The same basic principles that hold true for furniture at work - support

for your back, feet comfortably on the floor - are the same ones that should be employed at home.

Think firm enough that you can stand up out of it easily. Check out the furniture designs of the Scandinavian company, Ekornes. They design furniture for both beauty and comfort.

When you purchase, take your time. Sit on the chair or couch for about 20 minutes (which is about the length of time you should be sitting before you change positions anyway). How does your back feel? Can you stand up easily or does it require effort? Does the edge of the couch contact the back of your knees? Just as in the office chair, ideally there should be a 2-finger distance between your knees and the chair/sofa surface.

Lounge chairs are always a good choice. You can recline comfortably with good support for your neck and back.

Television
If you have a plasma television that is hung on the wall, hang it last. Position your furniture as you want it, then hang the television eye level, (while seated) so you are not looking up at it.

Telephone
Whether you use a home phone or a cell phone, NEVER support the phone between your ear and your neck. This tenses up the muscles of your neck and shoulders causing strain and pain.

Work Station
Same rules that apply for work at work apply for work at home. If you cannot have a dedicated workspace with a desk and ergonomic chair, set up your space so you are as neutrally aligned as possible. Don't do work in bed. Don't do work while lounging on the couch. Sit at a table on a chair with your feet on the ground. Change your position every 15 minutes, get up every 30 minutes.

Kitchen chairs/tables
I'm not such a stickler regarding kitchen chairs since they're usually used for short durations of time. But sometimes the kitchen is the place where people gather and commune even when there isn't eating involved. Look for a firm seat that doesn't come in contact

with the back of your knees, feet squarely on the floor and a full back.

Tables should be at a height where you can easily reach your plate without elevating your arms.

Sleeping

Beds, beds, beds!!! They are so subjective in terms of comfort. However, keep this in mind - think neutral alignment **always**. Neutral alignment is the position your head is in when you are walking around during the course of your day, head facing forward, ears over shoulders. This is one of the reasons stomach sleeping is frowned upon, it keeps your head rotated to one side.

Sleeping position

- **Back sleeper** - least amount of pressure on the back. Use pillows under your neck and knees to keep your back in good alignment.
- **Side sleeper** - follows sleeping on your back in terms of pressure on the spine. Use a pillow for your head as well as a pillow between your knees to maintain good spinal alignment. Your top leg should be even with or slightly behind your bottom leg with both knees bent.
- **Stomach** - is the least desirable position. It places a fair amount of stress on the back and the neck (your neck is in rotation over the course of the 5 - 7 hours that you sleep which contributes to neck stiffness and pain). If you must sleep on your stomach, place a pillow underneath your abdomen to encourage a neutral spine.

Mattresses

- Purchase a mattress that provides good back support and alignment.
- Stomach sleepers require firmer mattresses than back or side sleepers.
- Convoluted foam (which has an egg-carton appearance and feels soft yet resilient to touch) provides good support and comfort.
- Avoid coil mattress - they have little effect on quality or durability of mattresses.

- Specialty memory foams and custom options are not always the most comfortable, always try out mattresses for personal comfort.
- Mattresses have a life span of 8-10 years. Take care to replace them as they wear out

Pillows

Alignment of your head in relationship to your body is what should be kept in mind when you choose a pillow. When you are walking around during the day, your head is erect not bent to either side, flexed down towards your chest or looking up towards the sky. When you use a pillow, the same rules apply.

Stomach sleepers will have extreme rotation of the neck but should still maintain a position that is not side flexed.

Restfulness

I know people have different views on this but I'm going to share mine with you now.

Part of taking care of yourself involves resting your mind and body well. When it is time for you to sleep—SLEEP. Don't keep electronics in your bedroom.

Electronics + Bedroom = NO!!

There is evidence to suggest that the light from electronic devices interrupts sleep quality. Light, both indoor and outdoor, is a major synchronizer of your master clock.

Prior to the invention of electricity, the greatest degree of light exposure occurred between the hours of sunrise to sunset. These days we are exposed to more light during a 24-hour period and less darkness. This interferes with the group of cells in your brain called the superchiasmatic nuclei (SCN) which functions as your master clock.

These nuclei synchronize to the light-dark cycle of your environment when light enters your eye in conjunction with other biological clocks throughout your body.

Melatonin is a hormone that induces sleepiness. The brain begins to progressively increase the hormone around 9 pm or 10 pm and influences what time of day or night your body thinks it is no matter what time the clock says. When it is suppressed, there is less stimulation to promote sleepiness at a healthy bedtime. This means that people stay up later and miss valuable sleep and melatonin's potential health benefits (protection against cancer, diabetes, Alzheimer's disease and heart disease).

Light is measured in lux (trust me for keeping it simple here. It makes for a very interesting read if you want to learn more about light illumination but that's for another book).

To give you a few examples of light intensity:

Natural Light

10,752 Lux	Full daylight
1,075 Lux	Overcast day
107 Lux	Very dark day
10.8 Lux	Twilight
1.08 Lux	Deep Twilight
0.108 Lux	Full Moon
0.0108 Lux	Quarter Moon
0.0011 Lux	Starlight

Artificial Light

50 Lux	Cable tunnels, nighttime sidewalk, parking lots
100-150 Lux	Corridors, changing rooms, loading bay
200 Lux	Foyers, entrances, dining rooms, warehouses, restrooms
300 Lux	Libraries, sports and assembly halls, teaching spaces, lecture halls
500 Lux	Computer work, reading and writing, general offices, retail shops, kitchens
750 Lux	Drawing offices, chain stores, general electronics work
1000 Lux	Detailed electronics assembly, drafting, cabinet making, supermarkets
1500 – 2000+ Lux	Hand tailoring, precision assembly, detailed drafting mechanisms

Light from your computer screen or smartphone is enough to interfere with your circadian rhythm and melatonin production. Computer screens, smart phones and light bulbs emit blue light which eyes are particularly sensitive to since it's the type of light most common outdoors during daylight hours.

Melatonin is suppressed between 50 and 1000 lux. Compared with dim light, exposure to room light before bedtime suppressed melatonin, resulting in a later melatonin onset in 99.0% of individuals and shortening melatonin duration by about 90 min. Also, exposure to room light during the usual hours of sleep suppressed melatonin by greater than 50% in most (85%) trials.

However, the wavelength of light is very important here because red and amber lights do not suppress melatonin while blue, green and white lights do. If you must use an alarm clock in your bedroom, make sure the LEDs are red or amber.

Okay, that's some of the research. Now for what that means in terms of Oikonomics.

1. For committed couples, more intimate conversations without the interruption of television or laptop.

2. More conscious reflection to think about the day, to plan the coming day, or to meditate.

3. More SEX!!! Television in the bedroom = 50% less sex compared to those who do not keep a television in their bedroom.

4. Rooms have purpose - Kitchens are for cooking, dining rooms for eating, and OFFICES for working.

I was going to break this chapter down into various hobbies. Then I thought how complicated that would make things…for me. There are MILLIONS of hobbies but one through line.

Hobbies are usually passions. When you are immersed in your passion there is a loss of time. You began practice at 9am and it's now 4pm. I get it. I've been there. Here's the thing. When you are practicing, you are in one protracted position for a really, REALLY long time. It's the same as being at work. Your brain may know it's different, but your body doesn't. Set the timer and stretch. Period. I know you have to get your 10,000 hours in. You will. In better shape. If you move. I promise.;)

Traveling is like breathing. We do it every single day. The only thing that changes is the mode. I will address various modes of transportation, their potential problems and solutions.

Train/bus

Short duration trips—to and from work are normally not a problem. You are shifting in your seat, reading, playing with your phone, sleeping. If you happen to have an active back or neck problem then you may have to make adaptations.

Back pain - Take along a jacket or sweater, roll it up and place it behind your back which will give you more support for your lumbar spine.

Neck pain - Be careful how you are holding your head. Always think about being in a neutral position. If you are reading your Kindle, phone, newspaper or book, hold it in front of your face, not down in your lap.

Long duration trips consisting of several hours or days requires more awareness. Be sure you get up every hour; stretch and walk around if possible. While sitting, perform ankle pumps, butt squeezes, shoulder and neck circles. The point is - KEEP MOVING!

Planes

Ahhh, planes. The more we use them, the less comfortable they make them. Aside from the fact that leg room is becoming more and more scarce, the standard make and size of the seats has always been a problem. If you are of a more petite stature, the "head rest" which should be in line with the curve of your cervical spine ends up pushing your head forward which overtime, creates muscle fatigue and neck pain. Lumbar support is virtually nonexistent. If you are lucky enough to be on a plane that offers pillows and blankets gratis (forget that, you're paying for both in your fare), use the pillow to place behind your back and the rolled up blanket to place behind your neck.

Also, **keep moving**! Move your feet up and down; walk the aisle.

Cars

The way we get from our home to work and back again is frequently by car.

Seats - If they are bucket seats, immediately go out and purchase a lumbar support for your car. Bucket seats reduce the natural lordosis, (the forward curve) of your lumbar spine which creates pain and can facilitate the development of a herniated disc.

Posture - Select the proper height so your hips and knees are at 90 degrees and the proper distance from the wheel so you can utilize the entire seat as you drive. Be aware of leaning forward, keep your head and neck in a neutral position.

Long distance travel and blood clots

The reason I keep emphasizing the importance of movement is this, anyone traveling more than four hours at a clip, no matter the mode of transportation, can be at risk for developing blood clots or deep vein thrombosis (DVT).

Blood clots can form in the deep veins (veins below the surface that are not visible through the skin) of your legs during travel because you are sitting still in a confined space for long periods of time. The longer you are immobile, the greater is your risk of developing a blood clot. Many times the blood clot will dissolve on its own. However, serious health problems can occur when a part of the blood clot breaks off and travels to the lungs causing a blockage. This is called a pulmonary embolism, and it could be fatal. The good news is there are things you can do to protect your health and reduce your risk of blood clots during long-distance trips.

There are certain segments of the population who are at a greater risk of developing blood clots than others. Be more vigilant if you fall within the following categories:

- Older (risk increases after age 40)
- Obesity (body mass index [BMI] greater than 30kg/m2
- Recent surgery or injury (within 3 months)
- Use of estrogen-containing contraceptives (for example, birth control pills, rings, patches)
- Hormone replacement therapy (medical treatment in which hormones are given to reduce the effects of menopause
- Pregnancy and the postpartum period (up to 6 weeks after childbirth
- Previous blood clot or a family history of blood clots
- Active cancer or recent cancer treatment
- Limited mobility (for example, a leg cast)
- Catheter placed in a large vein
- Varicose veins

What are the symptoms of a Deep Vein Thrombosis?

Half of people with DVT have no symptoms at all. The following are the most common symptoms of DVT that occur in the affected part of the body, usually the arm or the leg.

- Swelling of your leg or arm
- Pain or tenderness that you can't explain
- Skin that is warm to the touch
- Redness of the skin

If you have any of these symptoms, contact your doctor immediately.

What are the symptoms of a Pulmonary Embolism?

You can have a PE without any symptoms of a DVT. Symptoms of a PE can include:

- Difficulty breathing
- Faster than normal or irregular heartbeat
- Chest pain or discomfort, which usually worsens with a deep breath or coughing
- Anxiety
- Coughing up blood
- Lightheadedness or fainting

If you have any of these symptoms, seek medical help immediately.

J oseph Hubertus Pilates was born in Monchengladbach Germany in 1883 to a naturopath mother and a prize-winning gymnast father. He was a sickly child, afflicted with asthma and rickets in addition to other ailments. Like Theodore Roosevelt (also born a sickly child) he turned to exercise and athletics to combat these ailments and studied various exercise techniques to expand his knowledge. He became enamored by the classical Greek ideal of a man balanced in body, mind, and spirit. He began to develop his own exercise system based on this concept.

As an adult, having rid himself of his childhood ailments, Joe Pilates became an avid skier, diver, gymnast and boxer.

In 1912 he went to England, where he worked as a self-defense instructor for detectives at Scotland Yard. At the outbreak of World War I, Joe was interned as an "enemy alien" with other German nationals. During his internment, Joe refined his ideas and trained other internees in his system of exercise. He rigged springs to hospital beds, enabling bedridden patients to exercise against resistance, an innovation that led to his later equipment designs (the Reformer). In 1918, an influenza epidemic struck England killing thousands of people. However, not a single one of Joe's trainees died. This, he claimed, testified to the effectiveness of his system.

Upon his release, Joe returned to Germany where his exercise method gained favor in the dance community, primarily through Rudolf von Laban, who created the form of dance notation most widely used today. Hanya Holm adopted many of Joe's exercises for her modern dance curriculum, and they are still part of the "Holm Technique." When German officials asked Joe to teach his fitness system to the army, he decided to leave Germany for good.

In 1926, Joe immigrated to the United States. During the voyage he met Clara Zeuner, whom he later married. Joe and Clara opened a fitness studio in New York, sharing an address with the New York City Ballet. Joe Pilates referred to his system of exercise as "Contrology" and his studio was called the "Studio for Body Contrology."

By the early 1960s, many of their clients were New York dancers. George Balanchine studied "at Joe's," as he called it, and also invited Pilates to instruct his young ballerinas at the New York City Ballet.

While dancers loved this method of exercise, Joseph created his system not for dancers, but for his own body and the bodies of the men with whom he was interned during WWI.

Over the years there were several students of Joe Pilates' methods that went on to teach his principles on their own:

Mary Bowen was a Jungian analyst who began teaching Pilates in 1975.

Ron Fletcher who opened a studio in Los Angeles in 1970 and attracted many Hollywood stars.

Eve Gentry was a dancer who taught Pilates in the early 1960s at NYU and later opened her own studio in Santa Fe, New Mexico.

Kathy Grant who was one of only two Pilates practitioners believed to have been officially certified by Joe (Lolita San Miguel was the other).

Jay Grimes studied with Joseph Pilates, with Joe's wife Clara, and with Joe's protégés Romana Kryzanowska and John Winters. In his 18 years as a professional dancer, he never suffered an injury, which he attributes entirely to Pilates.

Bruce King was a dancer who opened a studio in the mid-1970s in New York.

Romana Kryzanowska took over as director of the Manhattan studio around 1970 after Joe passed away.

Carola Trier was the only one of Joe's students to open her own studio while he was still alive with his explicit blessing.

Joe and Clara ran their "Studio for Body Contrology" for 50 years until his death at the age of 83.

The physical therapy mantra is "proximal stability for distal mobility." What this means is, the stronger your core or center, the more power is transferred through arms and legs. This is the basis for every activity imaginable.

Everyday acts from bending over to put on shoes, picking up a package, turning to look behind you, sitting in a chair, or just standing are just a few of the many mundane actions that rely on your core and that you might not notice until they become difficult or painful. Even basic activities of daily living (ADLs) like bathing or dressing engage your core.

Jobs that involve lifting, twisting, and standing, all rely on core muscles. But less obvious tasks, like sitting at your desk for hours, engage your core as well. Making phone calls, typing, using the computer, and similar work can make back muscles surprisingly stiff and sore, especially if you're not strong enough to practice good posture and aren't taking sufficient breaks.

Low back pain, a debilitating, sometimes excruciating problem affecting four out of five Americans at some point in their lives, may be prevented by exercises that promote well-balanced, resilient core muscles. When back pain strikes, a regimen of core exercises, coupled with medications, physical therapy, or other treatments are often prescribed for relief.

Golfing, tennis or other racquet sports, biking, running, swimming, baseball, volleyball, kayaking, rowing and many other athletic activities are powered by a strong core. Less often mentioned are sexual activities, which call for core power and flexibility, too.

Bending, lifting, twisting, carrying, hammering, reaching overhead, even vacuuming, mopping, and dusting are acts that spring from, or pass through, the core.

Your core stabilizes your body, allowing you to move in any direction, even on the bumpiest terrain, or stand in one spot without losing your balance. Viewed this way, core exercises can lessen your risk of falling.

Weak core muscles contribute to slouching. Good posture trims your silhouette and projects confidence. More importantly, it lessens wear and tear on the spine and allows you to breathe deeply. Good posture helps you gain full benefits from the effort you put into exercising, too.

For all of the reasons listed above, I recommend Pilates for my patients when it's time for discharge. Why? Because Joseph Pilates' philosophy was to strengthen your core, (what Joe Pilates referred to as your "Powerhouse" or "Girdle of Strength"), which consists of your abdominals, low back muscles, inner thigh muscles and buttocks, basically the muscles that support your spine.

Dr. Stuart M. McGill

Dr. Stuart M. McGill is a professor of spine biomechanics at the University of Waterloo in Ontario Canada.

After years of studying the spine, he came to the conclusion that the average sit up, with its repeated shearing and compression of the anterior vertebrae of the lumbar spine, over time, increased the possibility of a disc herniation.

Based on these findings, he developed an alternative to the basic sit up which is described on the following page. In addition to that, he describes his favorite core routine which I have termed, "The Power Core 4."

The Power Core 4

The McGill Sit up
Created to maintain the forward curve of the lumbar spine thus preventing anterior spinal compression.

- Lie on your back
- Keep one knee flexed and the other extended
- Place both hands in the small of your low back
- Without moving your neck, lift your upper body just high enough to clear both shoulders off the mat
- Exhale as you lift up, inhale as you return to the mat

Stir the Pot
If you have a physio ball, this is a great exercise to add to your core routine.

- Forearms on the physio ball
- Legs outstretched behind you wider than hip width apart to give you a triangular base of support
- Move your arms in a circular motion

The Side Bridge or Plank
- Place your right forearm on the mat
- One leg just in front of the other
- Lift your hips up, balancing on your forearm and feet
- Maintain alignment with your hip up towards the ceiling
- To take pressure off of the supporting forearm, cross your free arm in front of your chest
- Try holding for 15 seconds. Work up to 30 seconds
- Repeat on the other side

The Bird Dog
This is a physical therapy classic. The emphasis here is to keep the core as still as possible while moving the extremities into and out of position.

- Come into hands and knees position
- Point one arm in front of you and the opposite leg directly behind you (off the floor)
- Contract your abdominals and keep them contracted
- Hold for 10 seconds. Alternate.
- Repeat 10 times, each side counts as one

As I discussed previously, the core is not just about the abdominals but all of the structures that surround and support the spine which include the hip and low back muscles. This next group of exercises will definitely test your endurance and get you strong!

<u>**Power hips**</u>

Clamshell
- Lie on your side with your back and hips against the wall to ensure a stable position
- Bend your knees, your feet against the wall as well (no shoes!)
- While keeping your ankles together, lift your top knee up as high as possible (the wall will prevent your hips from moving out of alignment)
- Slowly return to starting position
- Repeat 15 to 30 times

Hip abduction
- Maintain the same position as described above
- Straighten out the top leg, keep it flush with the wall
- Slowly lift it up then down
- Repeat 15 - 30 times

Hip extension with slight abduction
- Turn onto your stomach
- Keep both legs straight
- Tighten your abdominals to prevent excessive lumbar extension
- Bring the working leg slightly out to the side
- While maintaining a fully straight leg, lift it up, then slowly lower
- Repeat 15 - 30 reps
- Repeat the circuit in reverse with the other leg

Bridges
- Lie on your back
- Bend both knees with your feet hip width apart
- Tighten your abdominals
- Tighten your glutes as you lift your hips up
- Hold for 3 seconds
- Slowly lower
- Repeat 15 - 30 times

Doing these activities is a great start to a strong core if you cannot participate in a regular Pilates class. If you want to do Pilates at home, there are numerous videos for you. I would suggest taking a few classes to get a good technique in place and getting a suggestion from the instructor for a video for independent use

F rom a lateral or sideways view, ideal posture shows earlobes over shoulders over hips over knees over ankles. Shoulders down, gently pinched back. Abdominals gently drawn in towards your spine in what in Pilates is called the abdominal scoop.

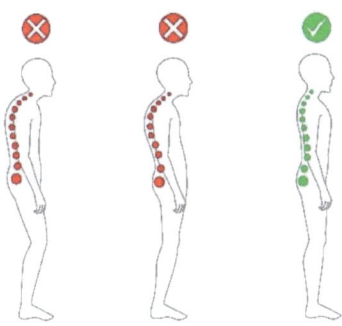

Elements of proper bending

Hips = hinge. All bending and leaning comes from the hips, <u>period</u>. There are no exceptions.

Examples:
- **Brushing teeth/washing your face** - When you are at the sink stick your butt out as you bend forward to spit, rinse or clean. If it feels weird or your significant other comes by and pinches it, you're doing it correctly.
- **Making the bed** - It's like tai chi - hinge at your hips and use your legs to gracefully move from side to side
- **Picking up from the floor** - Even if it's a piece of paper, hinge from your hips and bend your knees, I'm not kidding. I've treated many patients for back pain that struck when they "bent over to pick up a piece of paper." If you don't feel like going through all that trouble, utilize the golfer's pick up.

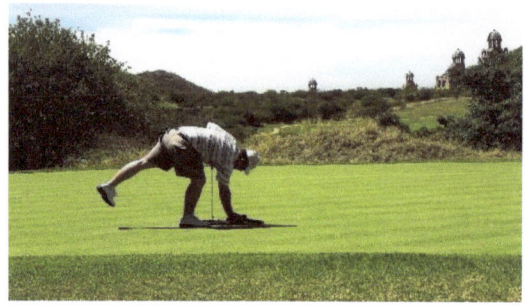

- **Picking up packages** - Hip hinge, knee bend, and abdominals tight. Keep package close to you. Stand up. Always do it this way, even if the box is empty. Repetition makes a habit. This is a habit that you want.

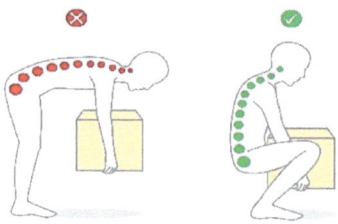

- **Sweeping/mopping** - This is another Tai Chi like movement pattern. Hinging at the hips, pushing and pulling to and fro with your legs, knees slightly bent. The danger is using your arms improperly which can result in tendinitis in your elbows or rotator cuff strain. Keep your arms outstretched as you hold the mop, broom. Use the strength of your legs to clean.

Neck
- Bring your right ear towards your right shoulder. Use your right hand to give a little over pressure. Hold for a count of 5
- Turn and look down towards your right hip. Bring your right hand slightly towards the back of your head. Hold for a count of 5. Repeat on the other side
- Look straight ahead. Gently give yourself a double chin. Return to your starting position. Repeat 10x

Shoulders
- Cross your right arm across your chest. Use your left hand to gently draw your right arm a little further. Hold for 5 seconds. Relax and repeat on the other side. Bring your right arm up over your head allowing your elbow to bend. Use your left arm to gently draw your right arm a little further. Hold for 5 seconds. Relax and repeat on the other side.

Back stretches
- Stand up and place your hands on your hips. Lean backwards. Hold for 5 seconds. Return to starting position. Repeat 5 times.

Wrists
- Bring your hands together as in prayer in front of your nose, elbows out. Keep your hands together, draw hands down towards your chest. Hold for 5 seconds.

Hips
- Stand up tall. Step forward with your right knee bent, keep your left leg straight. Tighten your butt muscles and your abdominals. Neither arch your back nor lean forward. Hold 5 seconds. Repeat on the other side.

Quadriceps
- Stand up tall. Bend your right knee. Take hold of your right foot with your left hand. Keep your knee facing straight down towards the floor. Don't arch your back. Hold for 5 seconds. Repeat other side.

Hamstrings

- Stand up. Place the heel of your foot on a chair. Keep leg straight and lean forward, from your hips. Hold for 5 seconds. Repeat other side.

Or

- While sitting straighten both legs in front of you, lean forward from your hips. Hold for 5 seconds.

Calf stretches

- Find a wall. Place both forearms the wall. Bring your left foot forward, bend your knee. Keep your right leg straight and your heel down. Lean into the wall. Keep your buttocks tight, your abdominals tight, don't arch your back. Hold for 10 seconds. Repeat other side

<u>Gentle strengthening exercises</u>

Glute sets

- Sit or stand. Clench your buttocks together, hold and relax. Repeat 10 times. (The beauty of these is nobody knows you are doing them!)

Scapular retractions (Shoulder blade squeezes)

- Stand or sit. Gently draw your shoulders down and back. Hold for 5 seconds. Repeat 10 times

Ankle pumps

- Keep both feet flat on the floor. Lift your heels up. Return to floor Lift your toes up. Return to floor. Repeat 20 times (each up and down is one repetition).

Contract Relax activity

- Beginning at your head and continuing sequentially through your entire body, contract and then relax every muscle you can. For example: Knit your brow then relax. Knit your brow and scrunch your nose. Relax both. Knit your brow, scrunch your nose and clench your teeth. Relax. Repeat this process until you are literally contracting every muscle in your body at the same time. This will help cue you in to tension spots when they crop up during your day. Do this in a quiet space without interruption.

References

History of Ergonomics. (n.d). Retrieved June 30, 2015, from
http://www.ergonomics-info.com/history-of-ergonomics.html

N Owen, A Bauman, W Brown. (December 9 2008). Too Much
Sitting: A Novel and Important Predictor of Chronic Disease Risk.
Br J Sports Med 43:81-83. Retrieved June 30, 2015, from
http://bjsm.bmj.com/content/43/2/81.full.pdf+html

How to Fit an Ergonomic Chair. (n.d.) Retrieved June 30, 2015, from
http://www.backdesigns.com/How-to-fit-an-ergonomic-chair.aspx

Porter, R (2013). CEAS I: Ergonomics Assessment Certification
Reference Manual. Atlanta, GA: The Back School

Sleep and Technology Don't Mix: Why You Need to Set an
Electronic Curfew. (n.d.). Retrieved August 5, 2015, from
http://articles.mercola.com/sites/articles/archive/2014/06/26/sleep-
electronic-gadgets.aspx

Reasons to Create a Technology Free Bedroom. (n.d.). Retrieved
August 6, 2015, from
http://www.becomingminimalist.com/technology-free-bedroom/

Office Ergo – Selecting a Chair. (n.d.). Retrieved August 6, 2015,
from http://ergonomics.ucla.edu/office-ergonomics/selecting-a-
chair.html

Measuring Light Levels. (n.d.). Retrieved August 7, 2015, from
http://sustainabilityworkshop.autodesk.com/buildings/measuring-
light-levels

Blood Clots and Travel: What You Need to Know. (n.d.) Retrieved
May 10, 2015, from http://www.cdc.gov/ncbddd/dvt/travel.html

I Gavish, B Brenner (April 6, 2011). Air travel and the risk of thromboembolism. Intern Emerg Med 2:113-6. Retrieved May 10, 2015 from http://www.cdc.gov/ncbddd/dvt/travel.html

Pilates Origins. (n.d.). Retrieved May 8, 2015 from http://www.pilates.com/BBAPP/V/pilates/origins-of-pilates.html

Who Was Joseph Pilates. (n.d.). Retrieved May 8, 2015 from http://www.JillianHessel.com

History of Pilates. (n.d.). Retrieved May 8, 2015 from https://pilatesology.com/faqs/history-of-pilates/

The Real World Benefits of Strengthening Your Core (n.d.). Retrieved May 9, 2015 from http://www.health.harvard.edu/healthbeat/the-real-world-benefits-of-strengthening-your-core

S McGill. (n.d.). Train the Core the Right Way. Retrieved June 10, 2015 from https://www.youtube.com/results?search_query=train+the+core+the+right+way

Recommendations

For those of you in NYC who need a physical therapist, massage therapist, acupuncturist or coach, I have compiled a list of places and people with whom I have had personal experience and trust. There are other resources that may be helpful to you in your quest for total wellness.

Physical Therapy
- Chelsea Physical Therapy
- Resolution Physical Therapy
- Yorkville Physical Therapy

Massage Therapy
- Exhale Spa
- Sherrin Bernstein, Touch Fitness & Attract Essentials
- American Massage Therapy Association

Acupuncture
- Olo Acupuncture
- Tri-State College of Acupuncture
- Pacific College of Oriental Medicine

Exercise Physiologists/Coaches
- Jonathan Cane, City Coach Multisport

Meditation/Spirituality
- Reverend Nafisa Shariff, Entering the Holy of Holies
- Tibet House
- Shambhala
- New York Insight Meditation

Back Care
- Relax The Back

Books
- *Stretching* by Bob Anderson
- *Why do I hurt?* by Adriaan Louw
- *Healing Back Pain: The Mind/Body Connection* by Dr. John E. Sarnow

Movement Therapies
- Alexander Technique
- Feldenkrais

Videos
- YouTube: Understanding Pain in Less than 5 minutes and what to do about it

About the Author

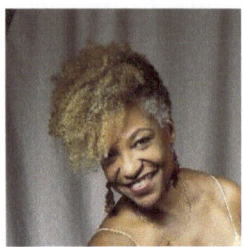

With a Bachelor's degree in physical therapy from SUNY Downstate Medical Center in Brooklyn and a diploma from New York's Swedish Institute of Massage Therapy as well a Certified Ergonomic Assessment Specialist designation from The Back School of Atlanta, Deidre Ann Johnson has been healing people with touch for over 20 years.

Her experience is varied, from the hospital setting and home care to outpatient orthopedics. It is in orthopedics, however, where she has acquired the most experience and in the field of ergonomics specifically, where she feels her true calling.

In addition to her career as a physical therapist, she is the co-author of *The Complete Idiot's Guide to Weight Training*; has completed a New York City Marathon (despite the fact that she HATED running) and was a two-time National and World Champion Powerlifter.

She resides in New York City with film maker Richard McKeown and her precious sweet pea kitty, Becky.

Appendix A

Sleeping with a neutral cervical spine

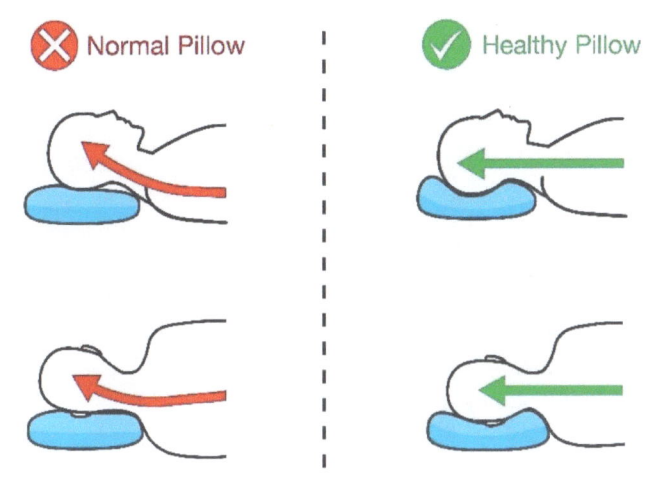

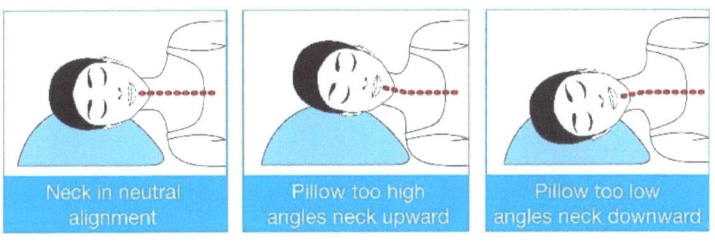

Appendix B

Neutral sleeping on your side (figure 1). Neutral sleeping on your back (figure 2).

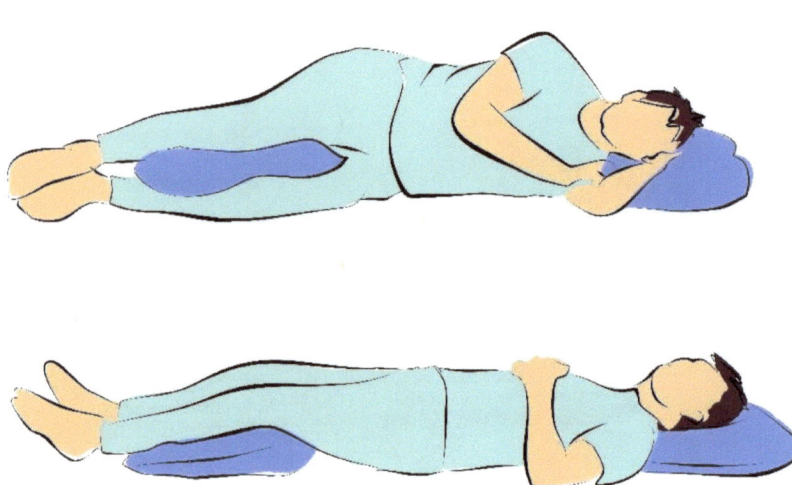

Appendix C

The spinal column

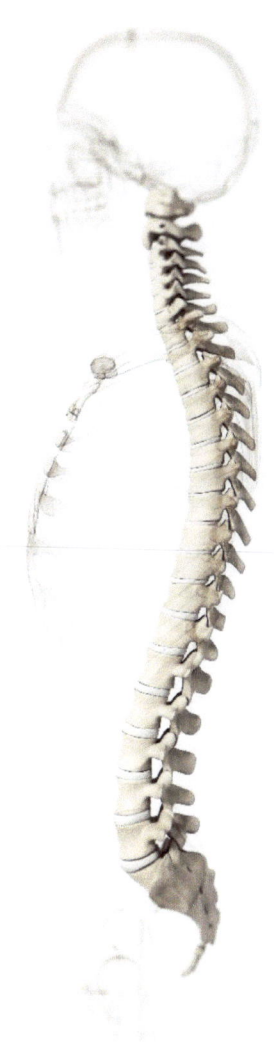

www.ingramcontent.com/pod-product-compliance
Lightning Source LLC
Chambersburg PA
CBHW050837290526
45792CB00001B/438